ALEX PARKER

The Smoothie Life

30 Recipes of Nutrient–Dense Ingredients to Reduce Inflammation, Boost Immune System, Decrease Sugar Cravings, and Fight Brain Fog

This book was professionally typeset on Reedsy.
Find out more at reedsy.com

"Let food be thy medicine, thy medicine
shall be thy food."

—Hippocrates

Contents

1

Introduction

Welcome to a journey into the vibrant world of smoothies where each sip brings you closer to wellness. This book isn't just a collection of recipes; it's an invitation to explore a lifestyle that's both delicious and nourishing. We're not just blending fruits and vegetables; we're creating recipes for a healthier, happier life. The power of smoothies is immense - they're not just delicious, but they also pack a punch when it comes to reducing inflammation, boosting your immune system, curbing sugar cravings, and clearing brain fog. Imagine waking up each morning feeling rejuvenated, both mentally and physically. This is the transformative power of the right nutrition.

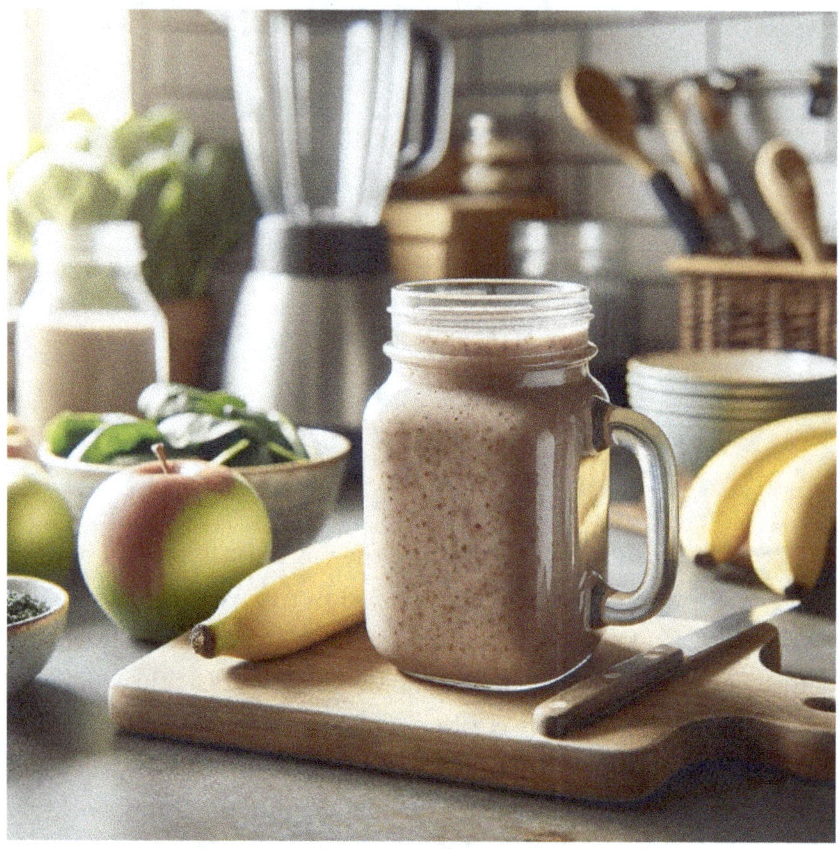

In our modern world, health challenges are prevalent, both in America and globally. Statistics paint a vivid picture of these issues. Obesity, for instance, is more than just about weight; it's a harbinger of various health complications, affecting approximately 42.4% of adults in the U.S. as of 2020. This is not just a number; it's a reflection of the struggles millions face daily with their health and wellbeing.

Inflammation, often a silent adversary, is at the heart of many health issues. It's like a fire within the body, sometimes burning unnoticed, leading to chronic diseases. Worldwide, chronic inflammatory diseases are a leading cause of death, with conditions like heart disease, cancer, and Type 2 Diabetes being prominent players in this arena. These diseases aren't just numbers; they represent real people dealing with real health battles every day.

Speaking of Type 2 Diabetes, it's a global concern, with an estimated 462 million individuals affected worldwide. The ripple effects of this condition are vast, impacting quality of life and longevity. Heart disease, too, takes a significant toll, being the leading cause of death globally, accounting for 16% of the world's total deaths.

Cancer, another major health challenge, has a profound impact, with an estimated 19.3 million new cancer cases and almost 10.0 million cancer deaths in 2020 alone. Each case is more than a statistic; it's a life, a family, a story.

These health issues are often exacerbated by our dietary choices. The average diet today is heavily skewed towards processed foods. In the U.S., ultra-processed foods contribute to 57.9% of total energy intake, while whole foods take a backseat. This preference for convenience over quality has far-reaching consequences for our health.

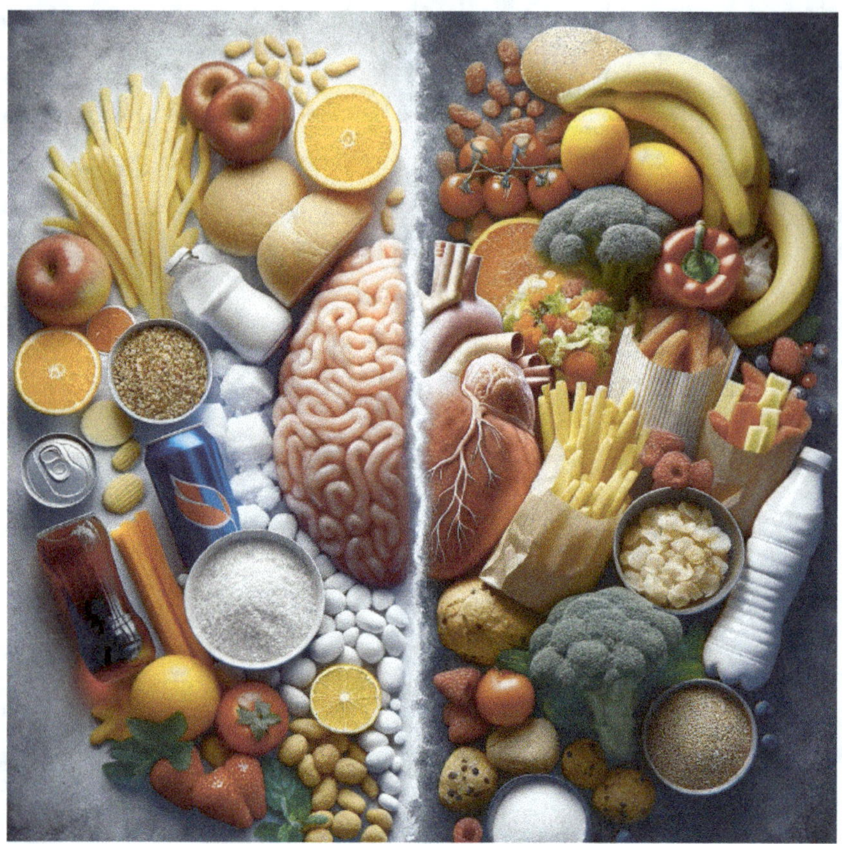

This book aims to be a beacon of change, guiding you towards a path where whole foods and natural ingredients take center stage. It's not just about recipes; it's about redefining your relationship with food and taking control of your health. So, let's turn the page and embark on this transformative journey together.

2

Preparation is Key

Welcome to Chapter 2, where we lay the foundation for your smoothie-making adventure. Preparation is not just a step; it's the key to making your smoothie journey effortless and enjoyable. Let's dive in!

5 Top Smoothie Blenders

First things first, the blender - your trusty sidekick in this journey. A good blender can make all the difference. We'll explore the top 5 blenders that cater to every need and budget, from the high-powered, multifunctional models to the compact, budget-friendly options. Each of these has its unique features, whether it's delivering silky smooth textures or being easy to clean, ensuring your smoothie-making is as smooth as the blend itself.

Vitamix 5200

- **Pros:**
- Powerful motor, perfect for blending even the toughest ingredients

into a smooth consistency.

- Large capacity container, ideal for making smoothies in bulk.
- Durable and long-lasting, with a reputation for reliability.
- Variable speed control for precise blending.
- **Cons:**
- Higher price point, making it a significant investment.
- Bulky design, requires more storage space.
- Louder operation compared to some other models.

Blendtec Total Classic Original Blender

- **Pros:**
- Extremely powerful, capable of blending a wide range of ingredients.
- Pre-programmed cycles for ease of use.
- Compact and modern design.
- Easy to clean with a self-cleaning feature.
- **Cons:**
- Also on the expensive side.
- The powerful motor can be quite loud.
- Some users may find the pre-programmed settings limiting.

Ninja Professional Countertop Blender (BL610)

- **Pros:**
- More affordable, offering good value for the price.
- Strong motor for its price range.
- Easy to use and clean.
- Large capacity, suitable for families or meal prepping.
- **Cons:**
- Less durable compared to high-end models.
- Can struggle with very hard or fibrous ingredients.

- The plastic jar might not feel as premium as glass or metal.

NutriBullet Pro

- **Pros:**
- Compact and ideal for small kitchens or personal use.
- Very easy to use and clean.
- Good for making single-serve smoothies.
- Affordable price point.
- **Cons:**
- Not suitable for large batches.
- Less versatile than larger, more powerful blenders.
- The motor may wear out faster with heavy use.

Oster Versa Pro Series Blender

- **Pros:**
- Powerful motor at a mid-range price.
- Durable with a stainless steel blade.
- Features pre-programmed settings and variable speed control.
- Comes with a tamper for processing thick mixtures.
- **Cons:**
- Bulkier than other mid-range models.
- The interface may not be as intuitive as other blenders.
- Some users report issues with the longevity of the plastic components.

Each of these blenders has its own unique strengths and potential drawbacks. Your choice will depend on your specific needs, preferences, budget, and how often you plan to use it for making smoothies.

* * *

Benefits of Meal Prepping

Meal prepping is like setting the stage for a week of healthy, hassle-free eating. It offers a multitude of benefits that can greatly enhance your daily routine and overall health. Let's delve into these benefits in more detail:

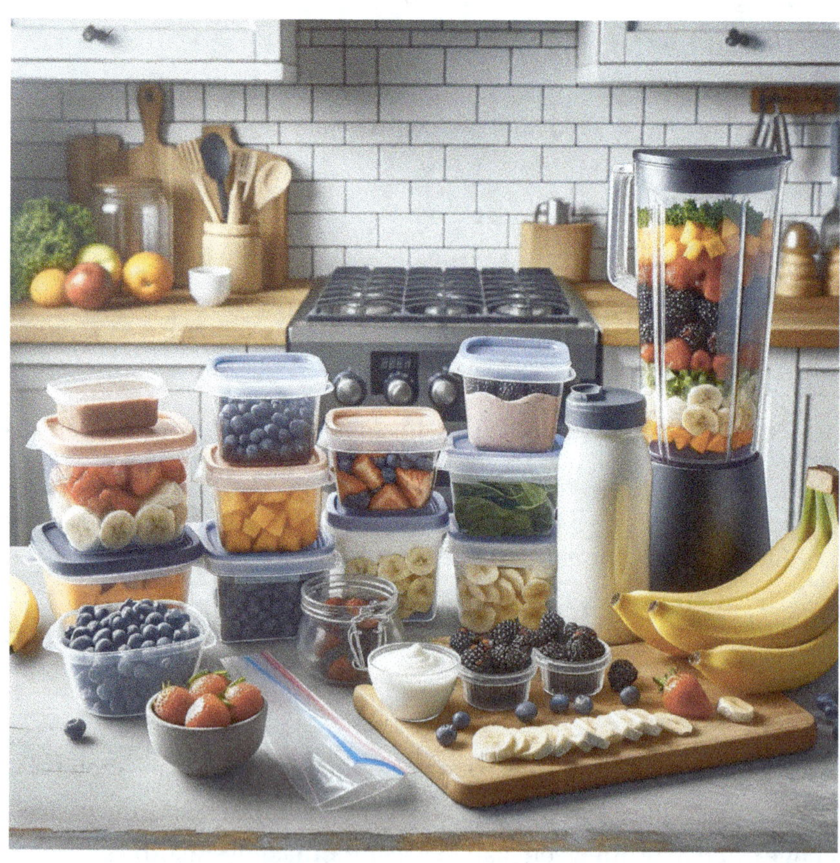

1. Saving Time:

One of the most immediate benefits of meal prepping is time efficiency. By dedicating a few hours to prepare your smoothie ingredients for the week, you save considerable time each day. Instead of starting from scratch for each smoothie, you simply grab your pre-prepped ingredients and blend. This streamlined process is particularly beneficial for busy mornings or when you need a quick nutritional boost without the hassle of extensive preparation.

2. Reducing Waste:

Meal prepping helps in reducing food waste significantly. By planning your smoothie ingredients in advance, you can buy exactly what you need and use it before it spoils. This approach not only minimizes waste but also encourages you to use every bit of the produce you buy. Additionally, when you prep and store your ingredients, such as chopping fruits and freezing them, you extend their shelf life, further reducing the likelihood of throwing food away.

3. Keeping Your Diet on Track:

For those focusing on maintaining a healthy diet, meal prepping is a game-changer. Prepping your smoothie ingredients in advance ensures that you have healthy options readily available, reducing the temptation to opt for less nutritious, convenient foods. It allows you to control what goes into your smoothies, helping you stick to specific dietary goals, whether it's increasing protein intake, reducing sugar, or ensuring a good balance of nutrients.

4. Variety and Creativity:

Prepping different combinations of fruits, vegetables, and supplements for your smoothies can add variety to your diet. This not only keeps your taste buds intrigued but also ensures a broader intake of nutrients. Experimenting with different recipes each week can be a fun and creative process, making your healthy eating routine more enjoyable.

5. Stress Reduction:

Knowing that your meals are planned and prepped in advance can significantly reduce mealtime stress. There's no last-minute decision-making or rush to prepare meals, which can be particularly relieving for those with busy schedules.

6. Cost-Effectiveness:

Meal prepping can also be more economical. Buying ingredients in bulk often costs less, and by planning your meals, you're less likely to make impulsive, expensive purchases. Furthermore, by utilizing all the food you buy, you get more value for your money.

In summary, meal prepping for smoothies not only saves time and reduces waste but also ensures that you maintain a healthy, varied, and enjoyable diet. It's a practical approach to eating that aligns well with a busy lifestyle, helping you stay on track with your health and wellness goals.

* * *

How-To Guide

Here's a step-by-step guide on how to efficiently prep your smoothie ingredients. This includes portioning fruits and vegetables, preparing smoothie packs, and organizing your ingredients for quick access. Meal prepping is not just about efficiency; it's about making healthy choices easy and convenient. This guide will help you streamline your smoothie-making process, ensuring you have quick and easy access to healthy, delicious smoothies any day of the week.

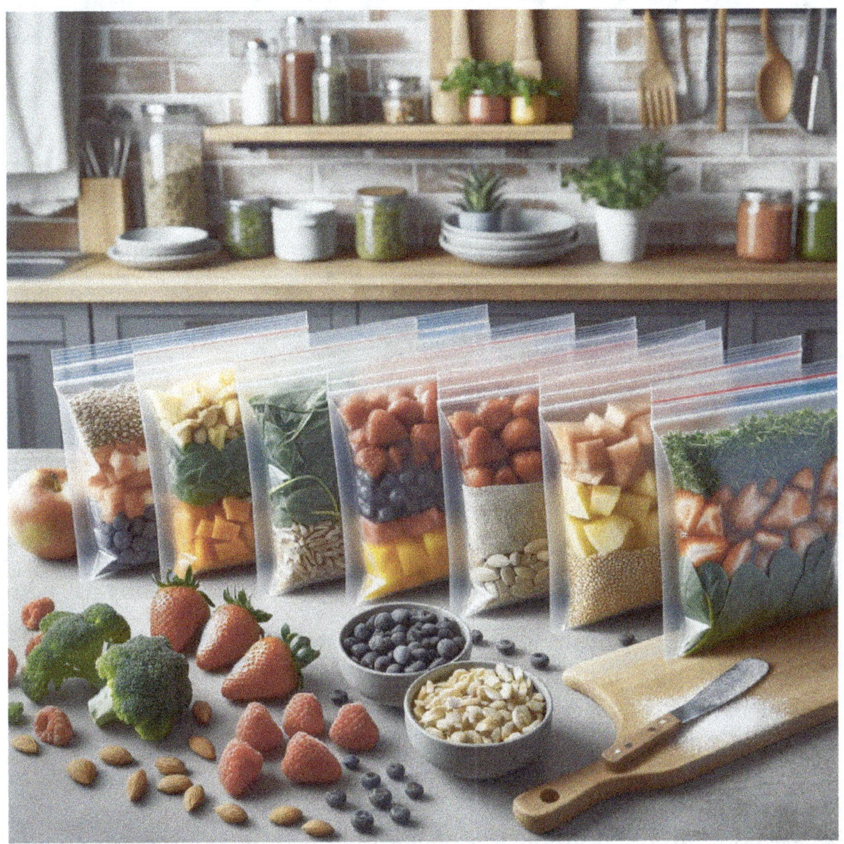

Step 1: Plan Your Smoothie Recipes

Start by deciding on the smoothie recipes you want to prepare for the week. This helps in determining the exact ingredients and quantities you'll need, ensuring a variety of nutrients and flavors.

Step 2: Shop for Ingredients

With your recipes in hand, make a shopping list of all the necessary fruits, vegetables, liquids (like almond milk, coconut water), and any add-ins (like protein powders, seeds, nuts). Buy in bulk where possible to save money, but be mindful of shelf life to avoid waste.

Step 3: Portion Fruits and Vegetables

Wash and dry all your fruits and vegetables thoroughly. Chop fruits and vegetables into blender-friendly sizes.

Step 4: Preparing Smoothie Packs

Create individual smoothie packs for each day of the week. Use ziplock bags or reusable silicone bags for this.

In each pack, combine the portioned fruits, vegetables, and any dry add-ins like seeds or nuts. Label each pack with the day of the week or the type of smoothie if you prefer variety.

Step 5: Freezing

Place your prepped smoothie packs in the freezer. This not only preserves their freshness but also means you can skip adding ice to your smoothies, as the frozen ingredients will chill the drink.

For ingredients that don't freeze well (like leafy greens or liquid bases), store them in the refrigerator or in a cool, dry place.

Step 6: Organize for Quick Access

Organize your freezer and refrigerator in a way that the smoothie packs and other ingredients are easily accessible. Keep them at the front or in a dedicated 'smoothie shelf'.Store your blender, cups, and any other equipment in an easily accessible place in your kitchen.

Step 7: Making Your Smoothie

When it's time to make your smoothie, simply grab a prepped smoothie pack from the freezer, add your liquid base and any additional ingredients that weren't frozen (like fresh greens or a scoop of protein powder), and blend until smooth.

Step 8: Enjoy and Clean Up

Enjoy your freshly made, hassle-free smoothie. Clean your blender and utensils immediately after use to avoid residue build-up.

This methodical approach to preparing your smoothie ingredients not only saves time but also ensures that you have a healthy option ready at all times. It simplifies your morning routine, reduces food waste, and keeps your diet diverse and nutritious. With everything prepped and at your fingertips, you're more likely to stick to healthy eating habits and enjoy a variety of delicious smoothies throughout the week.

* * *

Fresh vs. Frozen?

Fresh or frozen? That's a question many smoothie enthusiasts ponder. When it comes to smoothie preparation, choosing between fresh and frozen fruits and vegetables is a common dilemma. Both have their pros and cons, and understanding these can help you make informed decisions based on nutrition, taste, availability, and convenience.

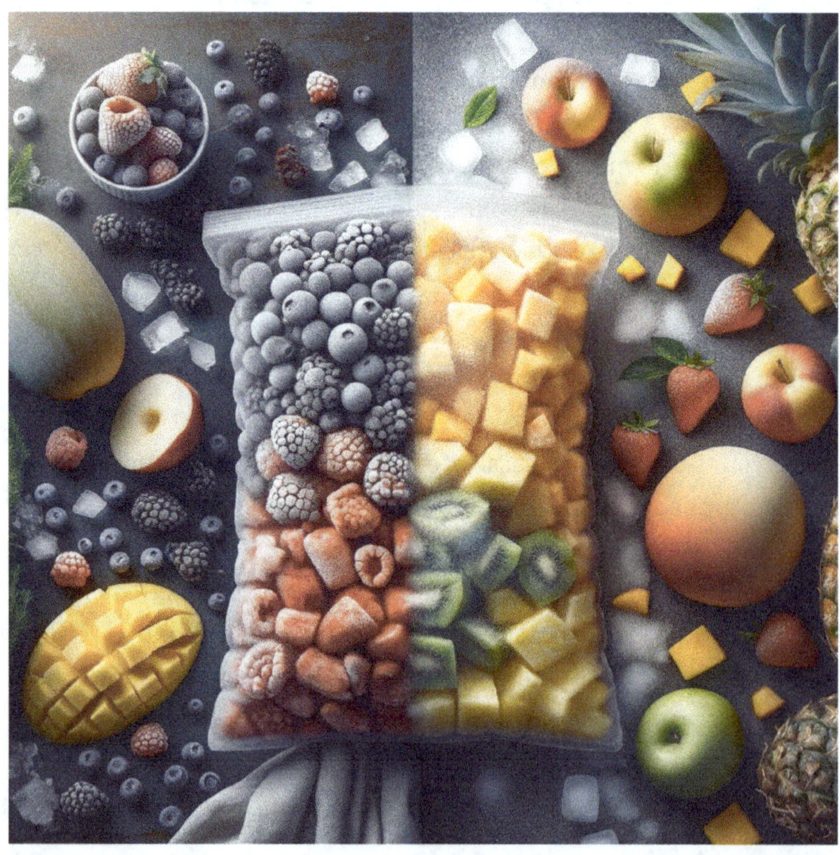

1. Fresh Fruits and Vegetables

Pros:

- **Taste and Texture:** Fresh produce often offers superior taste and texture. The crispness of fresh vegetables and the juiciness of fresh fruits are hard to beat, especially if they are in season.
- **Nutrient Content at Peak Ripeness:** When consumed at peak ripeness, fresh fruits and vegetables can have a higher nutrient content compared to some frozen options.
- **Variety:** Fresh produce provides a wide variety, especially seasonal items which can inspire a range of creative smoothie recipes.
- **Immediate Use:** Fresh fruits and veggies are ready to use without the need for thawing, making them convenient for immediate smoothie preparation.

Cons:

- **Shelf Life:** Fresh produce has a limited shelf life. They can spoil quickly, leading to waste if not used in time.
- **Availability:** Some fruits and vegetables are seasonal and may not be available year-round, or they might be more expensive off-season.
- **Preparation Time:** Fresh produce often requires more prep time — washing, peeling, chopping — before it can be used in a smoothie.

2. Frozen Fruits and Vegetables

Pros:

- **Convenience:** Frozen produce is pre-washed and pre-cut, which saves a lot of time in preparation.

- **Longer Shelf Life:** Frozen items can be stored for a longer period without spoiling, reducing food waste.
- **Nutrient Retention:** Freezing preserves the nutrients of fruits and vegetables. Often, they are frozen at peak ripeness, which locks in their nutritional value and flavor.
- **Year-Round Availability:** Frozen fruits and veggies are available throughout the year, regardless of the season, providing consistency in your diet.
- **Cost-Effective:** Generally, frozen produce can be more cost-effective, especially for out-of-season or exotic items.

Cons:

- **Texture Changes:** Freezing can alter the texture of some fruits and vegetables, making them less appealing when thawed.
- **Risk of Freezer Burn:** If not stored properly, frozen produce can suffer from freezer burn, which affects taste and quality.
- **Nutrient Loss in Blending:** Some studies suggest that blending frozen produce immediately from frozen can result in a slight loss of nutrients compared to fresh produce.

3. Making the Best Choice

The decision between fresh and frozen produce for your smoothies depends on several factors:

Seasonality: Opt for fresh fruits and veggies when they are in season for the best taste and nutrient content. In the off-season, frozen varieties are a great alternative.

Convenience: If you have a busy lifestyle, frozen produce can be a time-saver, whereas if you enjoy the prep work and have the time, fresh produce is a delightful option.

Budget: Consider your budget. Fresh, in-season produce can be economical, but for off-season items, frozen varieties may offer better value.

Dietary Goals: If you're aiming for maximum nutrient intake and you have access to fresh, ripe produce, it's a great choice. However, if you're looking for consistency and convenience without significant nutrient loss, frozen is an excellent option.

In conclusion, both fresh and frozen fruits and vegetables have their own set of advantages and drawbacks. Your choice can vary based on your personal preferences, lifestyle, and goals. Often, a mix of both fresh and frozen produce can be the best approach to enjoy a variety of nutrient-rich, delicious smoothies all year round.

* * *

Buying in Bulk and Where to Buy

Bulk buying can be a game-changer for regular smoothie drinkers. Buying in bulk not only helps your wallet but also ensures you always have smoothie ingredients on hand.

Buying ingredients for your smoothies in bulk offers several advantages, ranging from financial savings to environmental benefits. Here's an in-depth look at the benefits of bulk buying and some tips on where to find the best deals.

Benefits of Buying in Bulk

1. Cost Savings: Bulk purchasing typically comes with a lower price per unit. This means significant savings over time, especially for ingredients that you use regularly in your smoothies.

2. Ensuring Consistent Supply: Having a bulk supply means you're less likely to run out of essential smoothie ingredients. This is particularly helpful for non-perishable items like seeds, nuts, and powders.

3. Encourages Healthy Eating: When you have a stock of healthy ingredients readily available, you're more likely to stick to your smoothie routine and resist the temptation of less healthy options.

Finding the Best Deals

1. Local Farmer's Markets: Farmer's markets are excellent for fresh, seasonal produce. They often offer competitive prices and the opportunity to support local farmers. Buying in bulk directly from farmers can sometimes allow for negotiation on prices, especially towards the end of the market day.

2. Wholesale Clubs: Stores like Costco, Sam's Club, and BJ's offer a wide range of products in bulk, often at discounted prices compared to regular grocery stores. These clubs are ideal for stocking up on non-perishable items and frozen fruits and vegetables.

3. Online Retailers: Online stores can be a convenient option for bulk buying, especially for dry goods like seeds, nuts, and protein powders. Websites like Amazon, Thrive Market, or Bulk Foods offer competitive pricing and home delivery, saving you time and effort.

4. Community Supported Agriculture (CSA): Joining a CSA can be a cost-effective way to receive a regular supply of fresh, seasonal produce. It also fosters a connection with local farmers and provides insights into how your food is grown.

5. Bulk Bins in Grocery Stores: Many grocery stores have bulk bin sections where you can purchase the exact amount of dry goods you need. This is ideal for trying out new ingredients without committing to a large quantity.

Tips for Bulk Buying

1. Assess Your Needs: Before bulk buying, consider your consumption rate to avoid over-purchasing perishable items.

2. Storage Solutions: Ensure you have adequate storage space and proper containers to store your bulk purchases, especially for perishable items that might need to be frozen.

3. Stay Organized: Keep an inventory of what you have in stock to avoid unnecessary purchases and to use older items first.

4. Mind the Shelf Life: Be aware of the shelf life of products to use them at their peak quality.

In summary, buying in bulk can be a smart, cost-effective, and environmentally friendly approach to stocking up on smoothie ingredients. By choosing the right places to shop and being mindful of your storage and usage, you can make the most out of bulk buying for your smoothie preparations.

In this chapter, we're not just preparing ingredients; we're preparing you for a seamless, enjoyable smoothie-making experience. So, let's get prepped and ready to blend!

3

Supplements to Give You That Extra Boost

In Chapter 3, we explore the realm of supplements – those extra touches that can turn your smoothie from a simple beverage into a powerhouse of nutrition. Whether you're looking to enhance your protein intake, support joint health, or just boost your daily nutrient intake, the right supplement can make all the difference. Let's dive into the benefits of adding supplements to your smoothies and highlight some popular options along with their nutritional values.

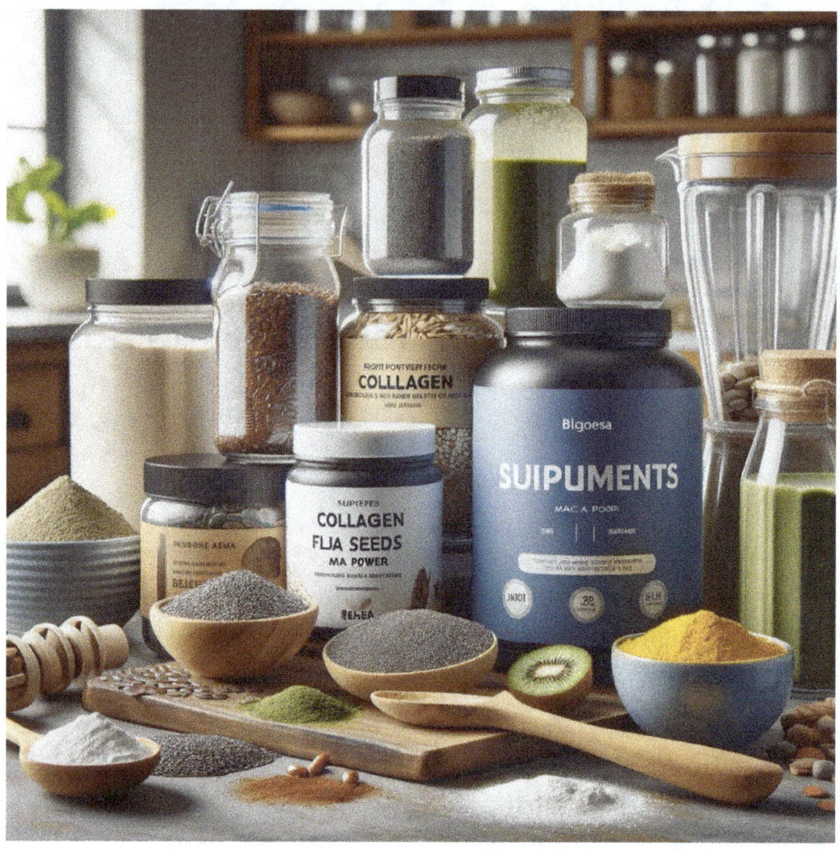

The Benefits of Adding Supplements to Your Smoothies

Adding supplements to your smoothies can significantly enhance their nutritional profile. Supplements can:

1. **Fill Nutritional Gaps:** They can provide vitamins, minerals, and other nutrients that you might not get enough of in your daily diet.
2. **Target Specific Health Goals:** Whether it's boosting protein intake for muscle repair or adding antioxidants for skin health, supple-

ments can be tailored to your specific health needs.

3. **Enhance Energy and Performance:** Certain supplements can increase energy levels, improve athletic performance, or aid in post-workout recovery.
4. **Convenience:** Supplements offer a convenient way to boost the nutritional value of your smoothies, especially on busy days.

List of Supplements and Their Nutritional Value

Protein Powder:

- *Benefits:* Supports muscle growth, repair, and maintenance. It's also key for bone health and maintaining a healthy metabolism.
- *Types:* Whey, casein (dairy-based), pea, hemp, brown rice, and soy (plant-based).
- *Nutritional Value:* High in protein, often enriched with other nutrients like vitamins and minerals.

Collagen:

- *Benefits:* Promotes skin elasticity, supports joint health, and may improve gut health.
- *Nutritional Value:* Rich in amino acids, particularly glycine, proline, and hydroxyproline.

Chia Seeds:

- *Benefits:* High in omega-3 fatty acids, fiber, and antioxidants. Great for digestive health and maintaining cholesterol levels.
- *Nutritional Value:* Good source of minerals like magnesium and calcium.

Flax Seeds:

- *Benefits:* High in omega-3 fatty acids, lignans (which have antioxidant properties), and fiber. Supports heart health and digestive health.
- *Nutritional Value:* Rich in protein and essential minerals.

Spirulina:

- *Benefits:* A blue-green algae packed with vitamins A, C, E, and B vitamins, and minerals like iron, magnesium, and potassium. Known for its detoxifying properties and boosting the immune system.
- *Nutritional Value:* High in protein and antioxidants.

Maca Powder:

- *Benefits:* Known for enhancing energy, stamina, and mood. Also believed to improve libido and hormone balance.
- *Nutritional Value:* Rich in vitamins and minerals, including vitamin C, copper, and iron.

Matcha:

- *Benefits:* High in antioxidants, specifically catechins. Boosts brain function and promotes heart health.
- *Nutritional Value:* Contains a unique set of amino acids and is a good source of EGCG (epigallocatechin gallate).

Turmeric (with Black Pepper):

- *Benefits:* Contains curcumin, a compound with strong anti-inflammatory and antioxidant properties. Black pepper increases its bioavailability.
- *Nutritional Value:* Anti-inflammatory, boosts brain-derived neurotrophic factor.

Cocoa/Cacao Powder:

- *Benefits:* Rich in polyphenols, which are antioxidants that promote heart health and may improve mood and symptoms of depression.
- *Nutritional Value:* Contains flavanols, magnesium, and iron.

Wheat Germ:

- *Benefits:* Excellent source of plant-based protein. High in fiber and omega-3 fatty acids. It contains antioxidants like selenium and Vitamin E, which bolsters the immune system and protects cells from damage caused by free radicals.
- *Nutritional Value:* High in vitamins and minerals including niacin, thiamine, and folate, which are essential for bodily functions. It provides important minerals such as zinc, magnesium, and iron.

Hemp Seeds:

- Benefits: Hemp seeds are a nutritional powerhouse, offering plant-based protein and a perfect balance of essential omega-3 and omega-6 fatty acids, beneficial for heart and brain health. They also possess anti-inflammatory properties, aiding in reducing chronic disease symptoms, and are high in fiber for improved digestion.
- Nutritional Value: Packed with protein, vitamins like vitamin E, and minerals such as phosphorus, magnesium, and zinc, hemp seeds

enhance overall health and nutrition.

Incorporating these supplements into your smoothies is not just about adding nutritional value; it's about enhancing your overall health and well-being in a delicious, convenient way. As you explore these supplements, remember to consider any dietary restrictions or allergies and consult with a healthcare provider if you have any health conditions or concerns.

In the next chapter, we'll journey into the world of detox smoothies, unveiling recipes that cleanse, rejuvenate, and revitalize.

4

The Power of a Detox

In Chapter 4, we delve into the rejuvenating world of detox smoothies. Embarking on a healthy eating journey often begins with resetting your system, and a detox smoothie cleanse can be an effective and delicious way to kick-start this process. Let's explore the benefits of beginning with a detox smoothie cleanse and then dive into a carefully curated list of detox smoothie recipes for a 3-day cleanse, complete with ingredient measurements.

Benefits of Starting with a Detox Smoothie Cleanse

A detox smoothie cleanse offers numerous benefits as a preamble to a healthy eating journey:

1. **Eliminates Toxins:** A detox cleanse helps in flushing out toxins accumulated due to processed foods, environmental pollutants, or unhealthy eating habits.
2. **Resets Digestive System:** These smoothies are packed with fiber and essential nutrients, aiding in resetting and soothing the digestive system.

3. **Boosts Energy Levels:** By eliminating sugar-laden and processed foods and replacing them with nutrient-rich smoothies, you can experience a natural energy boost.

4. **Enhances Nutrient Absorption:** A detox cleanse can prime your body for better absorption of nutrients from foods consumed post-cleanse.

5. **Promotes Healthy Habits:** Starting with a detox can set a positive tone for your healthy eating journey, making it easier to adopt and maintain healthier habits.

3-Day Detox Smoothie Cleanse

Below are detox smoothie recipes designed for a 3-day cleanse. Each day includes a different smoothie for breakfast, lunch, and dinner, providing a range of nutrients and flavors.

Day 1:

Morning Kickstart

- 1 cup spinach
- 1 small cucumber
- 1/2 green apple
- Juice of 1/2 lemon
- 1 tablespoon chia seeds
- 1 cup coconut water
- *Instructions: Blend all ingredients until smooth. This vibrant green smoothie is your perfect ally to kickstart the day with a burst of energy and hydration. Packed with spinach, cucumber, green apple, lemon juice, chia seeds, and coconut water, it's designed to refresh and revitalize your body from the first sip. *Use ice if not using any frozen ingredients.*

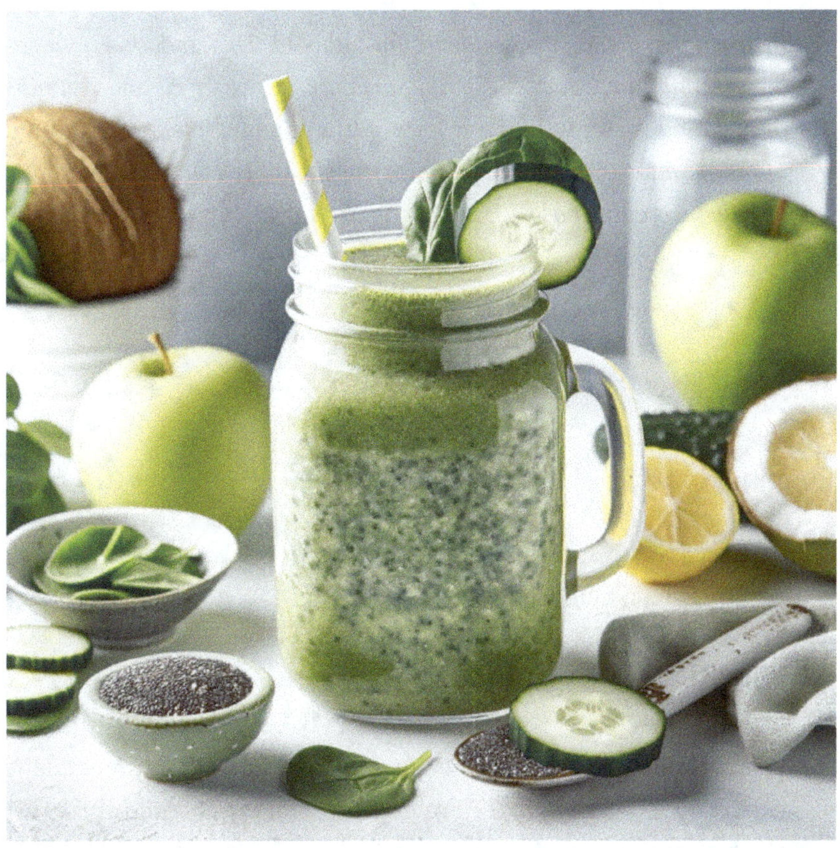

* * *

Midday Boost

- 1/2 beet, peeled and diced or canned
- 1 carrot, peeled and sliced
- 1/2 cup frozen pineapple chunks
- 1 teaspoon fresh ginger, grated
- 1 cup almond milk

- ***Instructions:*** *Blend all ingredients until smooth. This smoothie serves as a perfect midday boost, combining the natural sweetness and vitamins of beet and carrot with the tropical taste of pineapple. The addition of ginger adds a zesty kick and digestive benefits, while almond milk provides a creamy base. *Use ice if not using any frozen ingredients.*

* * *

Evening Soothe

- 1/2 avocado
- 1/2 cup frozen blueberries
- 1 tablespoon ground flaxseed
- 1 cup kale leaves
- 1 cup water
- ***Instructions:*** *Blend all ingredients until smooth. This smoothie is perfect for unwinding in the evening. The creamy avocado and sweet blueberries create a rich flavor, complemented by the nuttiness of ground flaxseed and the nourishing greens of kale. It's a soothing blend ideal for relaxation and nutrient replenishment. *Use ice if not using any frozen ingredients.*

* * *

Day 2:

Morning Refresh

- 1/2 cup strawberries
- 1/2 banana
- 1 tablespoon almond butter
- 1 teaspoon maca powder
- 1 cup oat milk
- **Instructions:** *Blend all ingredients until smooth. This smoothie is an excellent choice for a refreshing morning start. It combines the sweetness of strawberries and banana with the richness of almond butter and the energizing properties of maca powder, all smoothed together with oat milk for a deliciously creamy and nutritious breakfast option. *Use ice if not using any frozen ingredients.*

* * *

Midday Revitalize

- 1/2 cup frozen mango chunks
- 1/2 orange, peeled
- 1 small carrot
- 1 teaspoon turmeric powder
- 1 cup coconut water
- **Instructions:** *Blend all ingredients until smooth. This smoothie is ideal for a midday revitalization. It features mango and orange for a vibrant, citrusy sweetness, carrot for a dose of beta-carotene, and turmeric for its anti-inflammatory properties. Coconut water adds a tropical twist and ensures hydration, making this smoothie a refreshing, nutrient-rich pick-me-up. *Use ice if not using any frozen ingredients.*

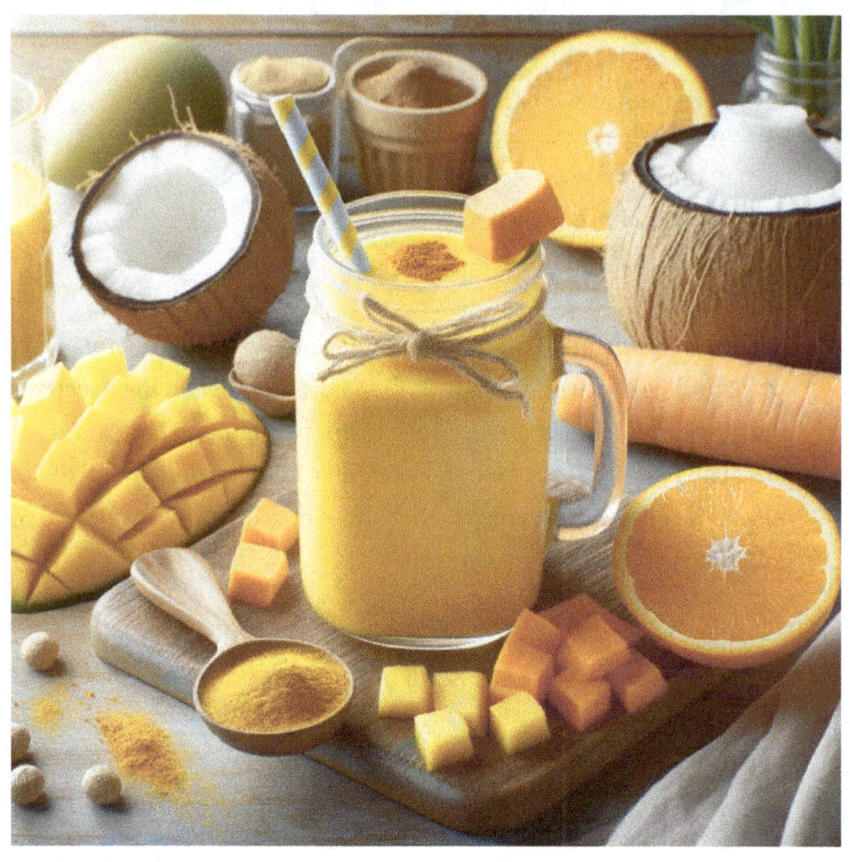

* * *

Evening Calm

- 1/2 cup sweet potato puree
- 1/2 pear
- 1 teaspoon cinnamon
- 1 cup spinach
- 1 cup almond milk

- **Instructions:** *Blend all ingredients until smooth. This smoothie is perfect for a soothing evening. The sweet potato puree and pear offer a gentle, comforting sweetness, complemented by the warmth of cinnamon. Spinach adds a nourishing touch, while almond milk creates a creamy, calming base, making it an ideal drink to unwind and relax before bedtime. *Use ice if not using any frozen ingredients.*

* * *

Day 3:

Morning Energize

- 1/2 cup frozen raspberries
- 1 small beet, fresh or canned
- 1 tablespoon cocoa powder
- 1 teaspoon chia seeds
- 1 cup water
- **Instructions:** *Blend all ingredients until smooth. This smoothie is a fantastic way to energize your morning. It combines the tartness of raspberries and the earthy flavor of beet with the richness of cocoa powder. Chia seeds add a boost of omega-3s and fiber, while water keeps the smoothie light and hydrating, perfect for kickstarting your day with vitality and flavor. *Use ice if not using any frozen ingredients.*

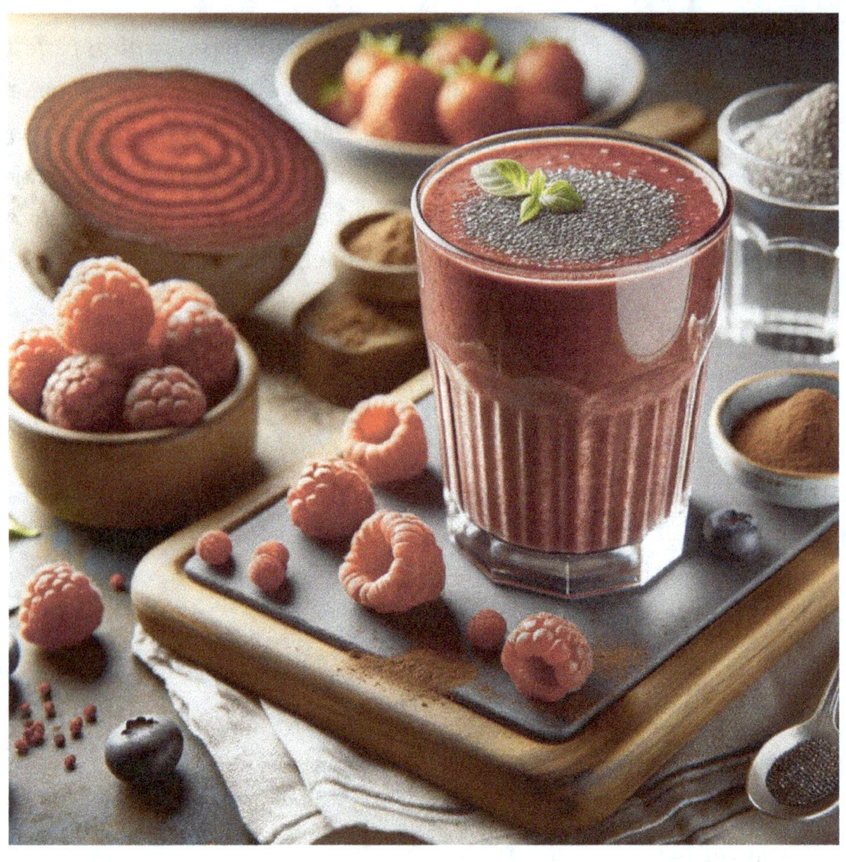

* * *

Midday Glow

- 1/2 apple
- 1/2 cup cucumber
- 1 stalk celery
- 1 tablespoon parsley
- 1 cup coconut water

- **Instructions:** *Blend all ingredients until smooth. This refreshing smoothie is perfect for a midday glow. It combines the crispness of apple and cucumber with the subtle earthiness of celery and the freshness of parsley. Coconut water adds a hydrating, tropical touch, making it an ideal choice for a nourishing and rejuvenating midday break. *Use ice if not using any frozen ingredients.*

* * *

Evening Harmony

- 1/2 cup pumpkin puree
- 1/2 banana
- 1 tablespoon hemp seeds
- 1 teaspoon ginger
- 1 cup oat milk
- **Instructions:** *Blend all ingredients until smooth. This smoothie is ideal for creating a sense of evening harmony. The pumpkin puree and banana offer a comforting, creamy base, complemented by the nuttiness of hemp seeds and the warm zing of ginger. Oat milk rounds out the smoothie, adding a soothing, creamy texture, perfect for a relaxing and nutritious end to your day. *Use ice if not using any frozen ingredients.*

* * *

These smoothies are designed to provide a balance of vitamins, minerals, antioxidants, and fiber. They are not only detoxifying but also flavorful and satisfying. During the cleanse, it's important to stay hydrated with plenty of water and herbal teas. Remember, a cleanse is a short-term reset, not a long-term diet solution. Always listen to your body and consult a healthcare professional if you have any health concerns.

As we turn the page to Chapter 5, we'll explore a wide array of smoothie recipes to sustain and enrich your healthy eating journey beyond the cleanse. Stay tuned for vibrant, nutrient-packed creations!

5

Anti-Inflammatory Recipes

I n Chapter 5, we delve into the heart of our smoothie journey - the anti-inflammatory smoothie recipes. These recipes are not just about tantalizing your taste buds; they are crafted to reduce inflammation in the body, boosts the immune system, decrease sugar cravings, and reduce brain fog, which is key to combating a host of health issues.

Inflammation is the body's natural response to protect itself against harm, but chronic inflammation can lead to various health issues. Anti-inflammatory smoothies, packed with ingredients like turmeric, ginger, berries, and leafy greens, provide a rich source of antioxidants and phytonutrients. These compounds help in reducing the production of pro-inflammatory cytokines and increase the production of anti-inflammatory cytokines. Regular consumption of these smoothies can help mitigate the effects of chronic inflammation, thus lowering the risk of diseases linked to it, such as arthritis, heart disease, and certain cancers.

A robust immune system is your first line of defense against infections and diseases. Ingredients commonly found in anti-inflammatory smoothies, such as citrus fruits, spinach, and nuts, are rich in vitamins C, E, and zinc, which play crucial roles in supporting the immune system. These nutrients help in the production and function of immune cells, providing a natural boost to your body's ability to fight off pathogens.

Regular consumption of sugary foods can lead to a cycle of highs and lows in blood sugar levels, which can increase cravings for more sugar. Anti-inflammatory smoothies can help break this cycle. By incorporating naturally sweet fruits and ingredients with low glycemic indices, such as apples, berries, and avocados, these smoothies provide a balanced blend of natural sugars and fibers. This helps in maintaining steady blood sugar levels, reducing the urge for sugary snacks. Additionally, the fiber in these smoothies increases satiety, keeping you fuller for longer and further helping to curb cravings.

Brain fog, characterized by confusion, forgetfulness, and lack of focus, can be exacerbated by poor diet, stress, and inflammation. Anti-inflammatory smoothies can play a role in alleviating these symptoms. Ingredients rich in omega-3 fatty acids (like flaxseeds and walnuts) and antioxidants (like blueberries and spinach) have been shown to enhance brain function. These nutrients help in reducing oxidative stress and improving blood flow to the brain, thereby enhancing cognitive functions and clearing brain fog.

In summary, anti-inflammatory smoothies offer a delicious and natural way to address some of the common health issues faced today. By carefully selecting ingredients that are known for their health benefits, these smoothies can significantly contribute to reducing inflammation, boosting immunity, curbing sugar cravings, and enhancing mental clarity, leading to improved overall health and well-being.

Each recipe combines ingredients rich in antioxidants, vitamins, and minerals to create delicious blends that soothe and nourish your body. Let's explore these carefully curated smoothie recipes designed to bring you health in every sip.

* * *

The Turmeric Sunrise

- 1 cup unsweetened almond milk
- 1/2 cup frozen pineapple chunks
- 1/2 banana
- 1/2 tsp turmeric powder
- A pinch of black pepper (to enhance turmeric absorption)
- 1 tbsp chia seeds
- ***Instructions:*** *Blend all ingredients until smooth. This smoothie is perfect for starting your day with a dose of anti-inflammatory turmeric, combined with the sweetness of pineapple and banana. *Use ice if not using any frozen ingredients.*

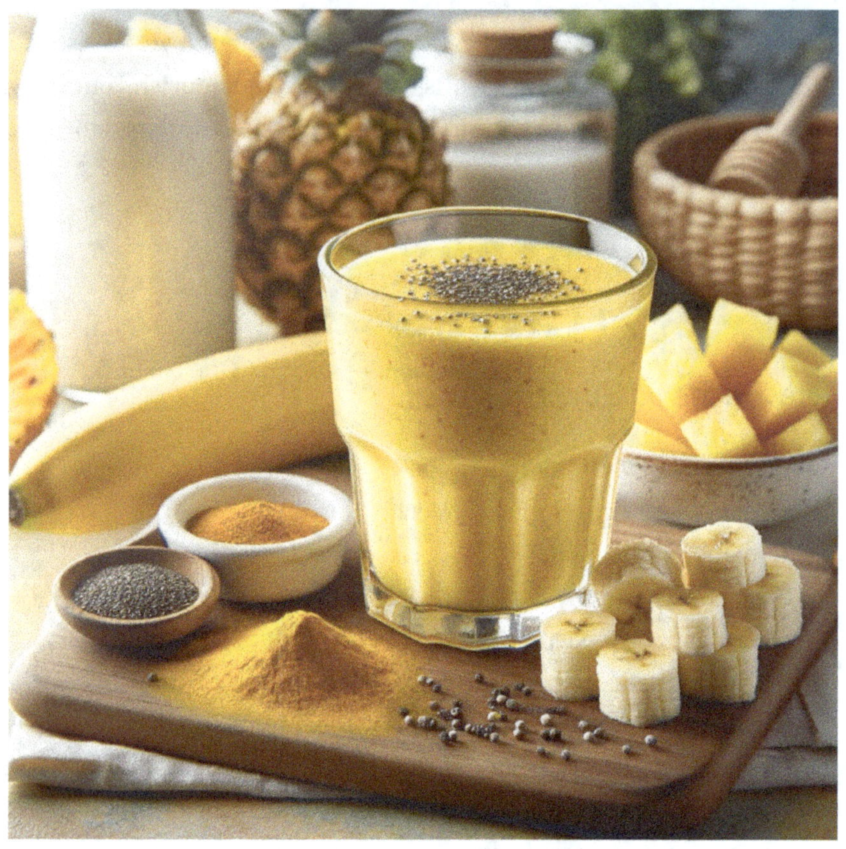

* * *

Green Ginger Glow

- 1 cup spinach
- 1/2 cup cucumber, chopped
- 1 small apple, cored and sliced
- 1/2 inch fresh ginger, peeled
- 1 tbsp flaxseed

- 1 cup coconut water
- **Instructions:** *Combine all ingredients and blend until smooth. This smoothie offers a refreshing mix of greens and ginger, a potent anti-inflammatory root. *Use ice if not using any frozen ingredients.*

* * *

Berry Omega Blast

- 1 cup frozen mixed berries (strawberries, blueberries, raspberries)
- 1/2 avocado
- 1 tbsp ground flaxseed
- 1 cup unsweetened oat milk
- A drizzle of honey (optional)
- **Instructions:** *Blend until creamy. This berry-rich smoothie is packed with omega-3 fatty acids from flaxseed and healthy fats from avocado. *Use ice if not using any frozen ingredients.*

* * *

Spicy Pineapple & Carrot

- 1 cup frozen pineapple chunks
- 1 carrot, peeled and sliced
- 1/2 inch fresh turmeric root or 1/2 tsp turmeric powder
- 1/4 inch fresh ginger root
- 1 cup water or coconut water

- **Instructions:** *Blend all ingredients for a tropical, anti-inflammatory treat with a spicy kick from ginger and turmeric. *Use ice if not using any frozen ingredients.*

* * *

Sweet Potato Cinnamon Soother

- 1/2 cup sweet potato puree or cooked
- 1/2 banana
- 1/4 tsp cinnamon
- 1 tbsp almond butter
- 1 cup almond milk
- **Instructions:** *Blend all ingredients until smooth. This smoothie is a comforting blend rich in anti-inflammatory properties and perfect for cooler days. *Use ice if not using any frozen ingredients.*

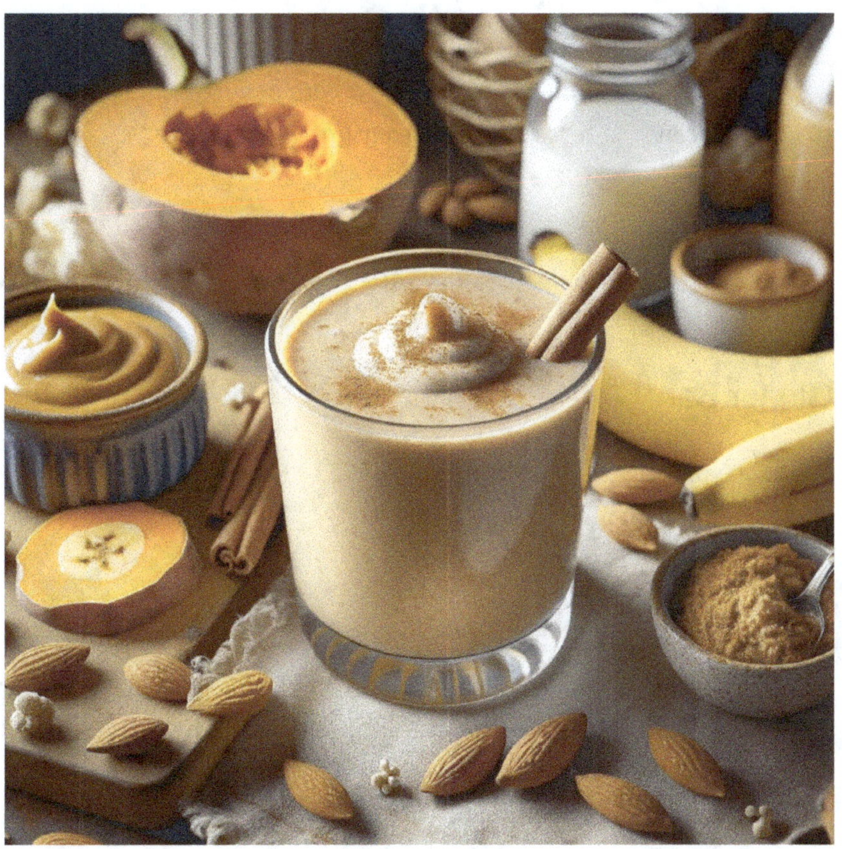

* * *

Kale Pineapple Detox

- 1 cup kale leaves
- 1/2 cup frozen pineapple chunks
- 1/2 apple
- 1 tbsp hemp seeds
- 1 cup water

- **Instructions:** *Blend until smooth. The kale and pineapple create a nutrient-dense, anti-inflammatory smoothie that's both detoxifying and delicious. *Use ice if not using any frozen ingredients.*

* * *

Ginger Berry Anti-Oxidant

- 1 cup spinach
- 1/2 cup frozen blueberries
- 1/2 cup frozen raspberries
- 1/2 inch ginger, peeled
- 1 tbsp chia seeds
- 1 cup almond milk
- **Instructions:** *Blend all ingredients until smooth. Enjoy the antioxidant benefits of berries and the soothing, anti-inflammatory effects of ginger in this refreshing smoothie. *Use ice if not using any frozen ingredients.*

* * *

Tropical Inflammation Tamer

- 1/2 cup mango, fresh or frozen
- 1/2 cup papaya
- 1/2 banana
- 1/4 tsp turmeric powder
- 1 cup coconut water

- **Instructions:** *Blend together for a tropical, anti–inflammatory treat. Mango and papaya add natural sweetness and aid in reducing inflammation. *Use ice if not using any frozen ingredients.*

* * *

Beetroot and Berry Blast

- 1 small beetroot, peeled and diced or canned beets
- 1/2 cup mixed berries
- 1/2 apple, cored and sliced
- 1 cup water
- 1 tsp lemon juice
- **Instructions:** *Blend all ingredients until smooth. Enjoy the detoxifying benefits of beetroot along with the antioxidants from berries in this vibrant smoothie. *Use ice if not using any frozen ingredients.*

* * *

Cherry Almond Anti-Inflammatory

- 1/2 cup tart cherries, fresh or frozen
- 1 tbsp almond butter
- 1/2 banana
- 1 cup spinach
- 1 cup almond milk
- **Instructions:** *Combine ingredients and blend until creamy. This*

*smoothie, rich in anti-inflammatory properties from cherries and almond butter, is both delicious and healthful. *Use ice if not using any frozen ingredients.*

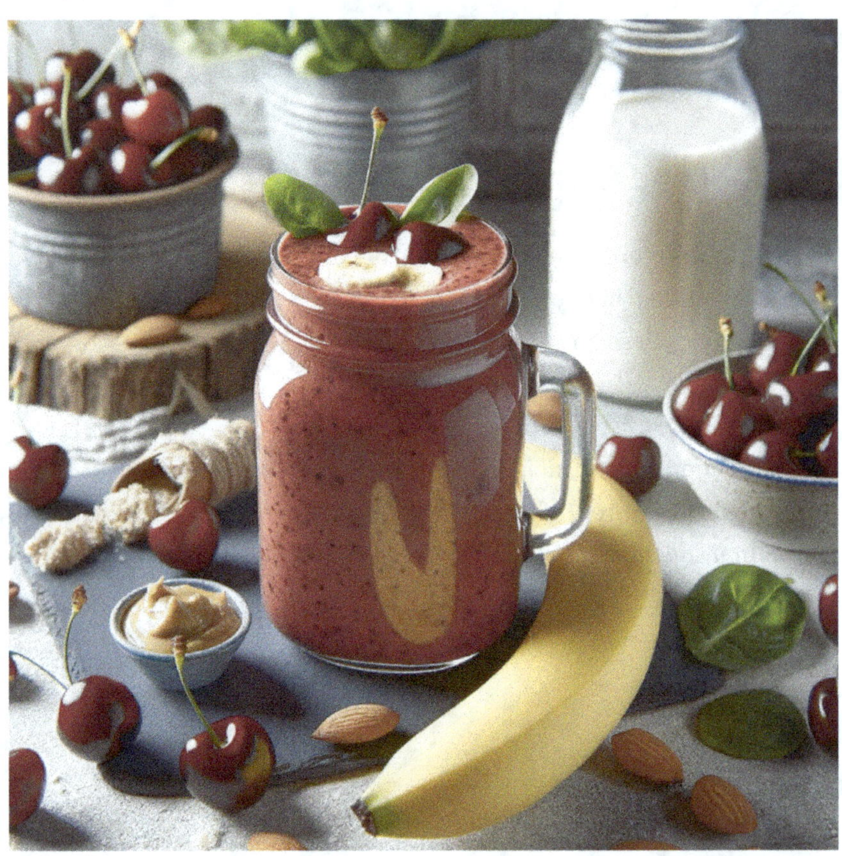

* * *

Avocado Green Machine

- 1/2 avocado
- 1 cup spinach
- 1/2 cucumber, chopped
- 1 tbsp hemp seeds
- 1 cup green tea (cooled)
- **Instructions:** *Blend all ingredients for a nutrient-rich green smoothie. Avocado and hemp seeds provide healthy fats, while green tea adds a dose of antioxidants. *Use ice if not using any frozen ingredients.*

* * *

Celery Refresh Tonic

- 2 stalks celery, chopped
- 1/2 green apple, cored and sliced
- Juice of 1/2 lemon
- 1 inch cucumber, chopped
- 1 cup water
- **Instructions:** *Blend together for a hydrating and refreshing smoothie. Celery and cucumber offer natural anti-inflammatory benefits. *Use ice if not using any frozen ingredients.*

* * *

Minty Melon Medley

- 1 cup watermelon, cubed
- 1/2 cup honeydew melon, cubed
- A handful of fresh mint leaves
- 1/2 lime, juiced
- 1 cup coconut water
- **Instructions:** *Blend all ingredients for a refreshing and hydrating smoothie. Watermelon and honeydew are great for inflammation, and mint adds a fresh twist. *Use ice if not using any frozen ingredients.*

* * *

Citrus Ginger Zinger

- 1 orange, peeled and seeded
- 1/2 grapefruit, peeled and seeded
- 1/2 inch ginger, peeled
- 1 tbsp honey
- 1 cup water
- **Instructions:** *Combine and blend until smooth. This citrus-packed smoothie is full of vitamin C and ginger, known for its anti-inflammatory properties. *Use ice if not using any frozen ingredients.*

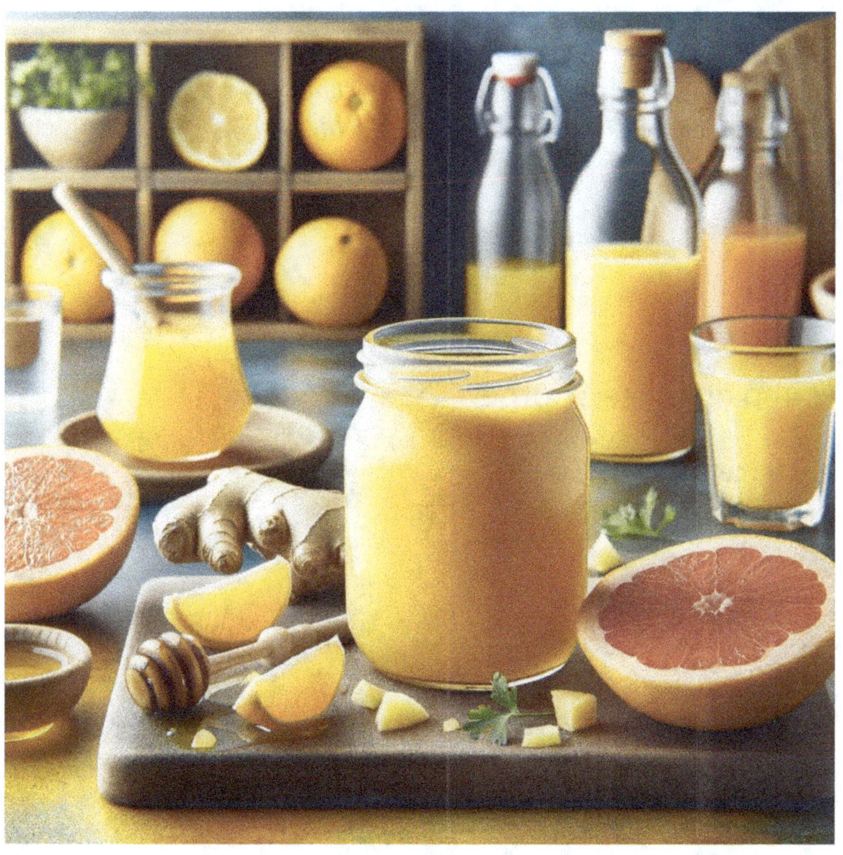

* * *

Blueberry Walnut Wonder

- 1 cup frozen blueberries
- 1/4 cup walnuts
- 1/2 banana
- 1 tbsp flaxseed meal
- 1 cup almond milk

- **Instructions:** *Blend together for a smoothie rich in antioxidants and omega-3 fatty acids. Blueberries and walnuts are excellent for fighting inflammation. *Use ice if not using any frozen ingredients.*

* * *

Pumpkin Spice Soother

- 1/2 cup pumpkin puree
- 1/2 banana
- 1/4 tsp cinnamon
- 1/4 tsp nutmeg
- 1 tbsp almond butter
- 1 cup oat milk
- **Instructions:** *Blend to enjoy a fall-inspired smoothie. Pumpkin is a great source of beta-carotene, and spices add anti-inflammatory benefits. *Use ice if not using any frozen ingredients.*

* * *

Pear and Spinach Detox

- 1 ripe pear, cored and sliced
- 1 cup spinach
- 1/2 cucumber, chopped
- 1 tbsp chia seeds
- 1 cup green tea (cooled)

- **Instructions:** *Combine all ingredients and blend. This green smoothie is perfect for detoxification and reducing inflammation. *Use ice if not using any frozen ingredients.*

* * *

Kiwi Kale Kickstart

- 2 kiwis, peeled
- 1 cup kale leaves
- 1/2 avocado
- 1 tbsp pumpkin seeds
- 1 cup water
- **Instructions:** *Blend for a nutrient–dense smoothie. Kiwi and kale provide a burst of vitamins, while avocado adds healthy fats. *Use ice if not using any frozen ingredients.*

* * *

Red Raspberry Rejuvenator

- 1 cup frozen raspberries
- 1/2 red bell pepper, chopped
- 1/2 apple
- 1/2 inch turmeric root, peeled
- 1 cup coconut water
- **Instructions:** *Blend together for an unusual but potent anti–inflammatory*

smoothie. *Red bell pepper and raspberries are high in antioxidants. *Use ice if not using any frozen ingredients.*

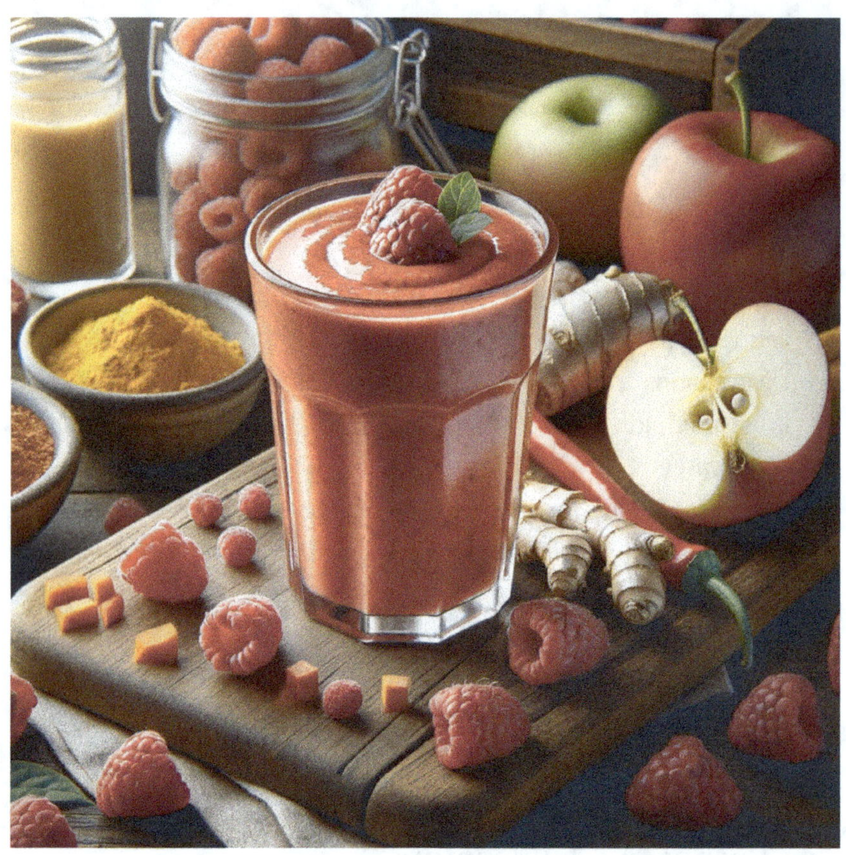

* * *

Carrot Cake Comfort

- 2 carrots, peeled and sliced
- 1/4 cup rolled oats
- 1/4 tsp cinnamon
- 1/4 tsp ginger powder
- 1 tbsp walnut pieces
- 1 cup almond milk
- **Instructions:** *Blend until smooth for a smoothie that tastes like dessert. Carrots and spices offer anti-inflammatory benefits. *Use ice if not using any frozen ingredients.*

* * *

Tropical Turmeric Temptation

- 1/2 cup mango chunks, fresh or frozen
- 1/2 cup frozen pineapple chunks
- 1/2 banana
- 1/2 tsp turmeric powder
- 1 cup coconut milk
- **Instructions:** *Combine and blend for a tropical smoothie with a turmeric twist. Mango and pineapple add sweetness and vitamins. *Use ice if not using any frozen ingredients.*

* * *

Berry Beet Bliss

- 1 small beet, peeled and diced or canned beets
- 1/2 cup strawberries, fresh or frozen
- 1/2 cup blueberries, fresh or frozen
- 1 tbsp hemp hearts
- 1 cup water
- **Instructions:** *Blend all ingredients for a vibrant and nourishing smoothie. Beets and berries are excellent for detox and reducing inflammation. *Use ice if not using any frozen ingredients.*

* * *

Soothing Cucumber Mint

- 1 cup cucumber, chopped
- A handful of fresh mint leaves
- 1/2 green apple, sliced
- 1 tbsp lemon juice
- 1 cup water
- **Instructions:** *Blend all ingredients for a refreshing and soothing smoothie. Cucumber and mint are excellent for hydration and reducing inflammation. *Use ice if not using any frozen ingredients.*

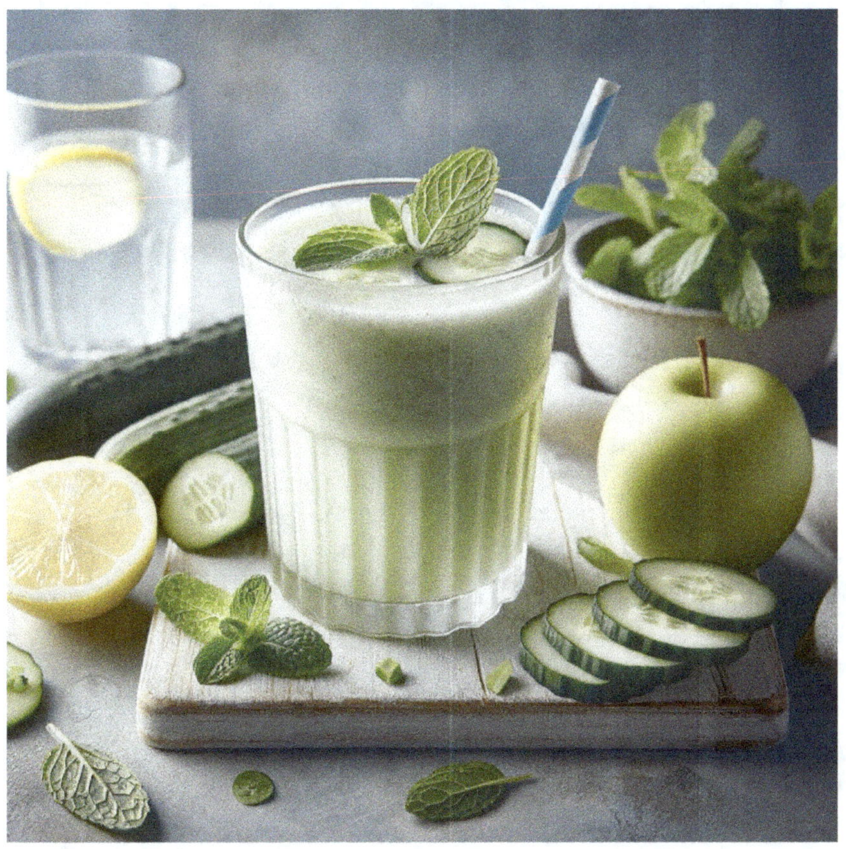

* * *

Spiced Sweet Potato Delight

- 1/2 cup sweet potato puree or cooked
- 1/2 tsp cinnamon
- 1/4 tsp nutmeg
- 1 tbsp maple syrup
- 1 cup almond milk

- **Instructions:** *Blend until creamy for a nutrient-rich, spiced smoothie. Sweet potatoes are loaded with vitamins, and spices add anti-inflammatory benefits. *Use ice if not using any frozen ingredients.*

* * *

Apple Ginger Reviver

- 1 green apple, cored and sliced
- 1/2 inch ginger, peeled
- 1 tbsp flaxseed meal
- 1 cup spinach
- 1 cup coconut water
- **Instructions:** *Combine and blend for a zesty and invigorating smoothie. Apple and ginger are great for digestion and inflammation. *Use ice if not using any frozen ingredients.*

* * *

Tropical Avocado Bliss

- 1/2 avocado
- 1/2 cup frozen pineapple chunks
- 1/2 cup mango chunks, fresh or frozen
- 1 tbsp lime juice
- 1 cup water
- **Instructions:** *Blend all ingredients for a creamy tropical smoothie.*

*Avocado adds healthy fats, and tropical fruits are rich in vitamins. *Use ice if not using any frozen ingredients.*

* * *

Zesty Carrot Orange

- 2 carrots, peeled and sliced
- 1 orange, peeled and seeded
- 1/2 inch turmeric, peeled
- 1 tbsp honey
- 1 cup water
- **Instructions:** *Blend to enjoy a bright and zesty smoothie. Carrots and oranges provide a boost of vitamins, and turmeric adds anti-inflammatory properties. *Use ice if not using any frozen ingredients.*

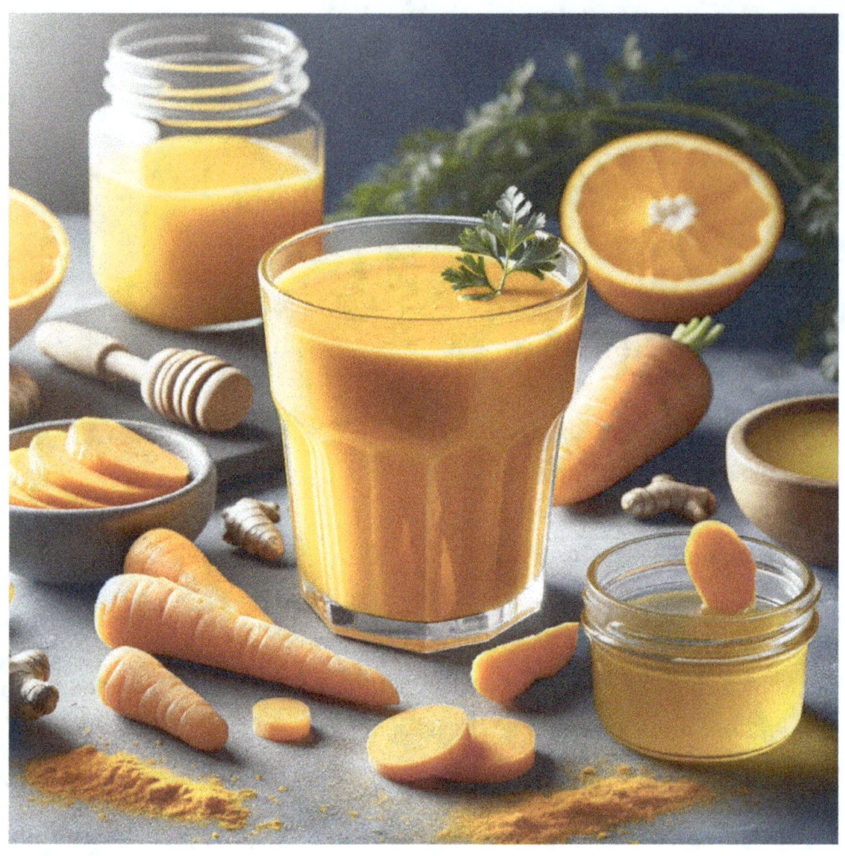

* * *

Pomegranate Berry Fusion

- 1/2 cup frozen pomegranate seeds
- 1/2 cup frozen mixed berries
- 1/2 banana
- 1 tbsp chia seeds
- 1 cup almond milk

- **Instructions:** *Combine and blend for a powerful antioxidant-rich smoothie. Pomegranate and berries offer a wealth of health benefits. *Use ice if not using any frozen ingredients.*

* * *

Peachy Kale Dream

- 1 cup kale leaves
- 1 ripe peach, sliced or frozen peaches
- 1/2 banana
- 1 tbsp ground flaxseed
- 1 cup almond milk
- **Instructions:** *Combine ingredients and blend for a smooth and dreamy smoothie. Peaches add natural sweetness, and kale is a nutrient powerhouse. *Use ice if not using any frozen ingredients.*

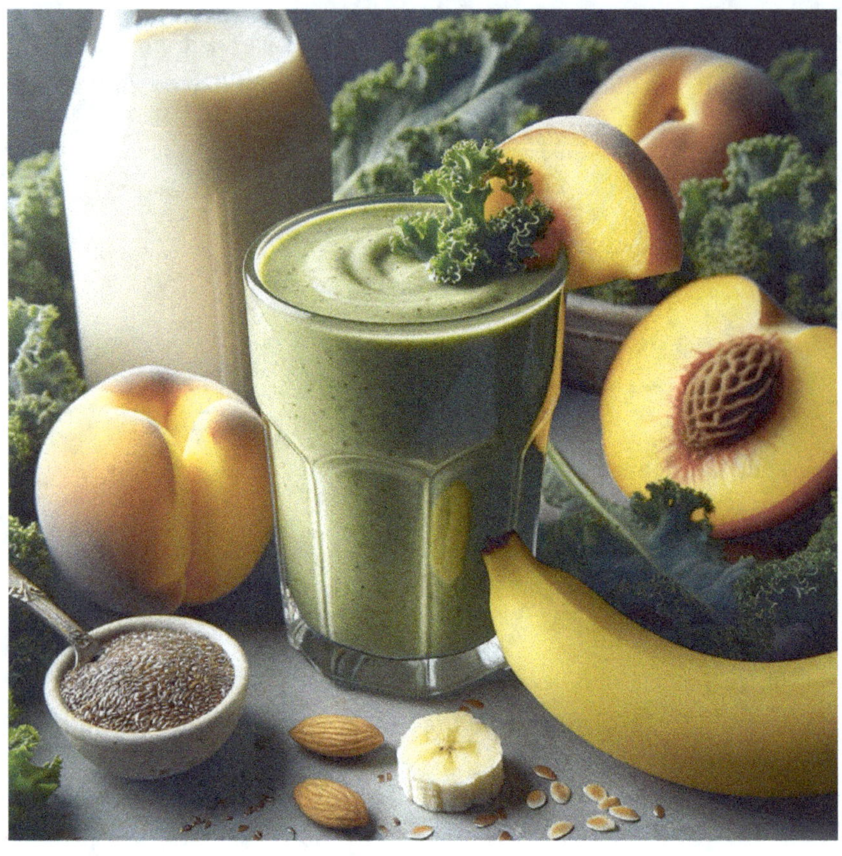

* * *

Cherry Spinach Supreme

- 1/2 cup tart cherries, fresh or frozen
- 1 cup spinach
- 1/2 avocado
- 1 tbsp hemp seeds
- 1 cup water

· **Instructions:** *Blend to create a rich and nourishing smoothie. Tart cherries and spinach are great for fighting inflammation, while avocado adds creaminess. *Use ice if not using any frozen ingredients.*

* * *

Each of these recipes brings a unique combination of flavors and health benefits. They are designed to be easy to prepare, making it simple for you to incorporate these anti-inflammatory powerhouses into your daily routine. Remember, the key to reaping the full benefits is consistency and variety – the more regularly you include them in your diet, the more you'll reap their anti-inflammatory benefits.

Enjoy these smoothies as part of a balanced diet, and feel the difference in your body and mind! Feel free to experiment with your own combinations using anti-inflammatory ingredients.

6

Embracing the Smoothie Lifestyle

As we reach the conclusion of our smoothie journey, it's time to reflect on the key points we've explored and the wealth of benefits that these delightful concoctions bring to our lives. This book has not just been about recipes; it's been a guide to adopting a healthier, more vibrant lifestyle through the power of smoothies.

1. **The Power of Ingredients:** We've seen how carefully selected ingredients can transform our health. From the anti-inflammatory properties of turmeric and ginger to the heart-healthy fats in avocados and hemp seeds, each component in our smoothies serves a purpose. They work in harmony to provide our bodies with essential nutrients, boost our immune systems, and help combat chronic inflammation.

2. **Diversity and Enjoyment:** The variety of recipes showcased in this book demonstrates that health and pleasure can go hand in hand. Whether it's the energizing "Morning Kickstart" or the soothing "Evening Calm," each smoothie offers a unique blend of flavors and health benefits, ensuring that your journey to wellness is never dull.

3. Ease and Practicality: We've emphasized the importance of preparation and practicality. Meal prepping, choosing the right blender, and understanding the balance between fresh and frozen ingredients are all part of making smoothies an easy and enjoyable part of your daily routine.

4. Nutritional Understanding: Through each recipe, we've gained insights into the nutritional benefits of different foods. This knowledge empowers us to make informed choices about what we consume, not just in our smoothies but in our overall diet.

5. A Holistic Approach: Ultimately, these smoothies are more than just drinks; they represent a holistic approach to health. They remind us that taking care of our bodies is a delicious adventure, one that can have profound effects on our physical and mental well-being.

As we close this book, remember that each smoothie you make is a step towards better health. The journey doesn't end here; it evolves with every blend, every taste, and every nourishing sip. Embrace the smoothie lifestyle, experiment with ingredients, and most importantly, enjoy the journey to a healthier you.

Your Feedback Matters: If you found this book beneficial and would like to support our journey together, please consider leaving a review on Amazon. Your feedback not only helps us but also guides others in their quest for health and wellness. Share your experiences, favorite recipes, and how this book has impacted your smoothie journey. Thank you for being a part of this flavorful adventure!

7

References

OpenAI. (2024). ChatGPT (GPT-4). OpenAI. https://chat.open
ai.com/

Furman, D., Campisi, J., Verdin, E., Carrera-Bastos, P., Targ,
S., Franceschi, C., Ferrucci,
L., Gilroy, D. W., Fasano, A., Miller, G. W., Miller, A. H., Mantovani, A.,
Weyand, C. M.,
Barzilai, N., Goronzy, J. J., Rando, T. A., Effros, R. B., Lucía, A.,
Kleinstreuer, N., &
Slavich, G. M. (2019). Chronic inflammation in the etiology of disease
across the life
span. *Nature Medicine*, 25(12), 1822–1832. https://doi.org/10.1038/s41
591-019-0675-0

Khan, M. A., Hashim, M., King, J., Govender, R. D., Mustafa, H., & Kaabi,
J. A. (2019).
Epidemiology of Type 2 Diabetes – Global burden of disease and
Forecasted Trends.
Journal of Epidemiology and Global Health, 10(1), 107.

https://doi.org/10.2991/jegh.k.191028.001

Steele, E. M., Baraldi, L. G., Da Costa Louzada, M. L., Moubarac, J., & Mozaffarian, D.
   (2016). Ultra-processed foods and added sugars in the US diet: evidence from a
   nationally representative cross-sectional study. *BMJ Open*, 6(3), e009892.
   https://doi.org/10.1136/bmjopen-2015-009892

Sung, H., Ferlay, J., Siegel, R. L., Laversanne, M., Soerjomataram, I., Jemal, A., & Bray, F.
   (2021). Global Cancer Statistics 2020: GLOBOCAN estimates of incidence and mortality
   worldwide for 36 cancers in 185 countries. *CA: A Cancer Journal for Clinicians*, 71(3),
   209–249. https://doi.org/10.3322/caac.21660

Trust for America's Health. (2023, February 6). *The State of Obesity 2020: Better Policies for
   A Healthier America - TFAH*. TFAH. https://www.tfah.org/report-detail s/state-of-
   obesity-2020/

Wartzman, E. (2024, January 12). 11 Best Blenders 2024. *The Strategist.*
   https://nymag.com/strategist/article/best-blenders.html

World Health Organization: WHO. (2020, December 9). *The top 10 causes of death.*
   https://www.who.int/news-room/fact-sheets/detail/the-top-10-cau ses-of-death